A Yoga Journey through Peru

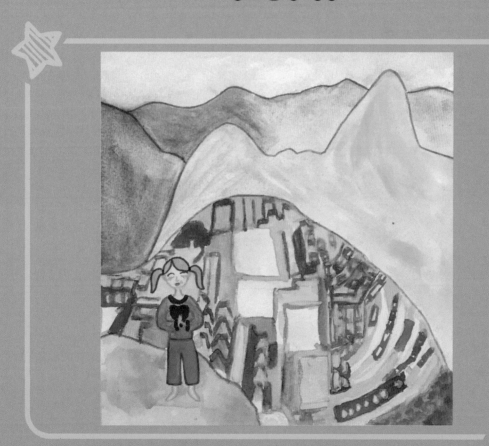

Amanda Marie Cottrell

Library of Congress Cataloging-in-Publication Data Available

ISBN: 978-1-7751434-3-7

Published by Art Mindfulness and Creativity

www.artmindfulnessandcreativity.com

Dedication:

For my daughter Ella, you teach me how to enjoy the precious moments of each day. For all the students I have ever taught, may you find joy in the mindful moments of life, and for all my fellow yogis, I love to practice and learn from you.

AMC

Hola, me llamo Ella! That means 'hello my name is Ella' in Spanish. Today we are going on a yoga adventure through the country of Peru. Peru is on the continent of South America and the official language is Spanish. Many people also speak Quechua and Aymara because they are the languages of the first people who lived there, the Incas.

Easy Pose/ Sukhasana
Sit criss cross with your hands at prayer center. Take a breath in and lengthen your spine nice and tall. Repeat a few times until you feel grounded and connected to your body

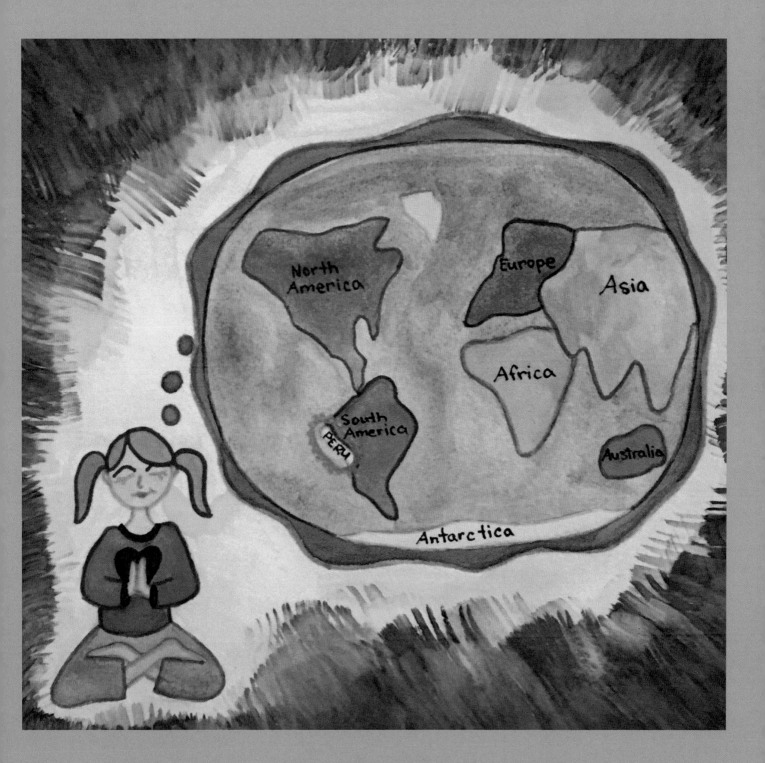

We have been asked to help find an Ancient Inca treasure that has been stolen from 'el Museo de Minerales' (The Museum of Minerals) in Lima. To get to Peru, we are going to take a magical balloon ride all the way to Lima, the capital city of Peru. To start our journey we will then need to fly from Lima to the Ancient Inca capital city, Cuzco.

Balloon Breath

Continue to sit criss cross and begin to focus on your breathing. As you inhale fill your belly up with air and lift your arms to the sky, imagine your belly is a balloon filling to a count of 4. As you exhale allow your balloon to deflate and lower your arms back by your sides to a count of 4. Repeat 5 times.

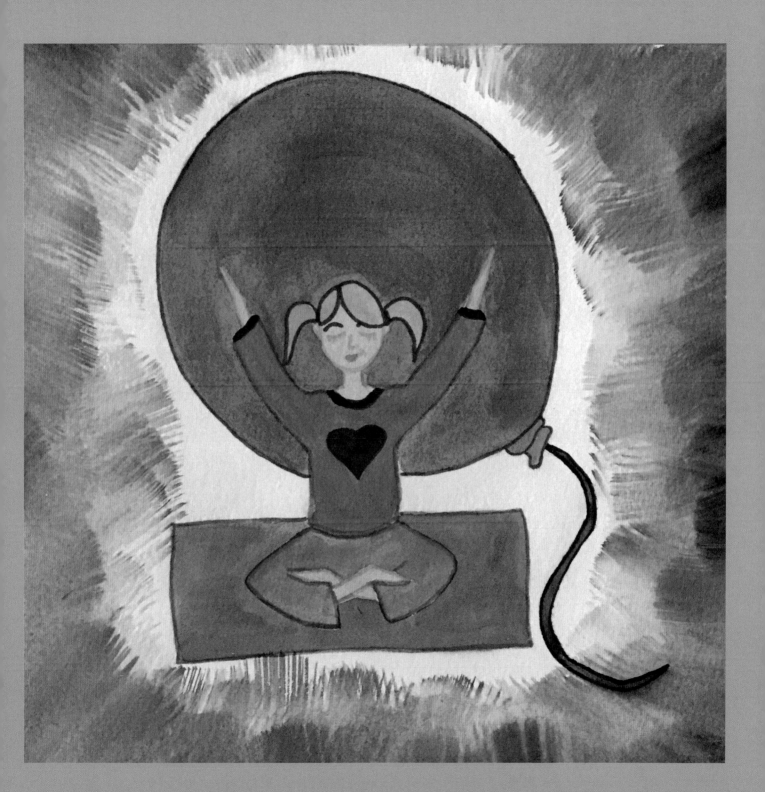

To find the treasure we are going to travel through Peru. On our quest we may come across some Peruvian animals like the jaguar, who lives in the Amazon Rainforest, and llamas, who live in the Andes Mountains. Did you know that llamas are cousins to the Vicuña? The Vicuña are so important to Peruvian culture that they are represented on their national flag.

Cat Cow/ Marjariasana

Lean forward onto your hands and knees and come into a tabletop position. Arch your back up to the sky like an angry jaguar then lower your belly and tilt your head up to the sky to be a Vicuna. Breathe out as you arch your back and inhale as you lower your belly. Repeat at least three more times.

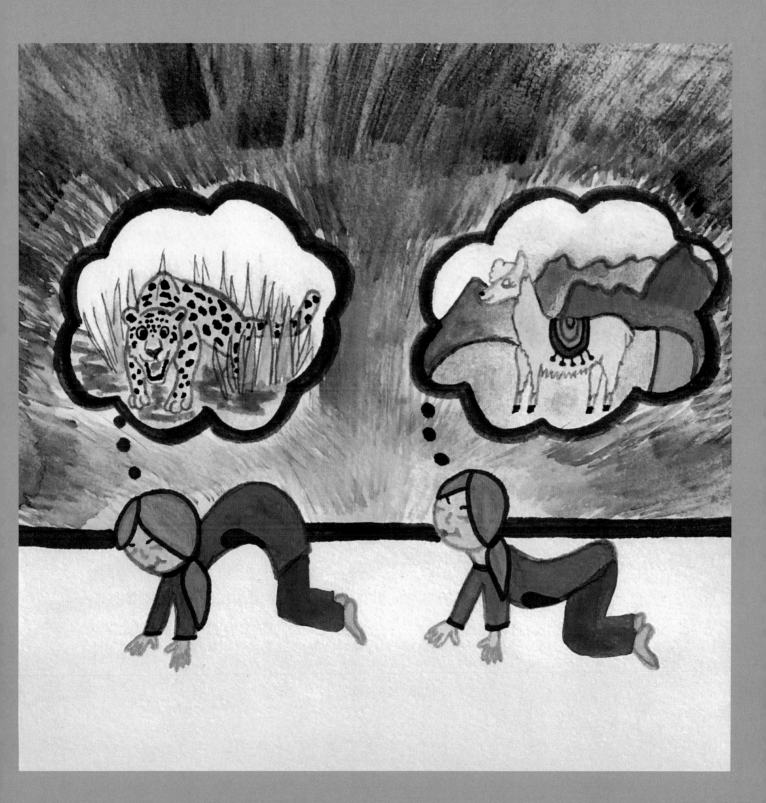

Since we are in Cuzco our adventure starts in the Andes Mountains. This mountain range spans 7 countries. It is the starting point of the Amazon River and holds the worlds largest mineral deposits. They mine for copper, gold and silver. The Andes Mountains also help feed the planet, both potatoes and tomatoes originated here. There are over 3,800 different types of potatoes grown in Peru's Andes Mountains.

Down Dog/ Adho Mukha Svanasana
Push your hips up to the sky like a great big mountain. Stretch out your legs and feel them grounding you to the earth. Hold for a few breaths then step forward to the top of your mat.

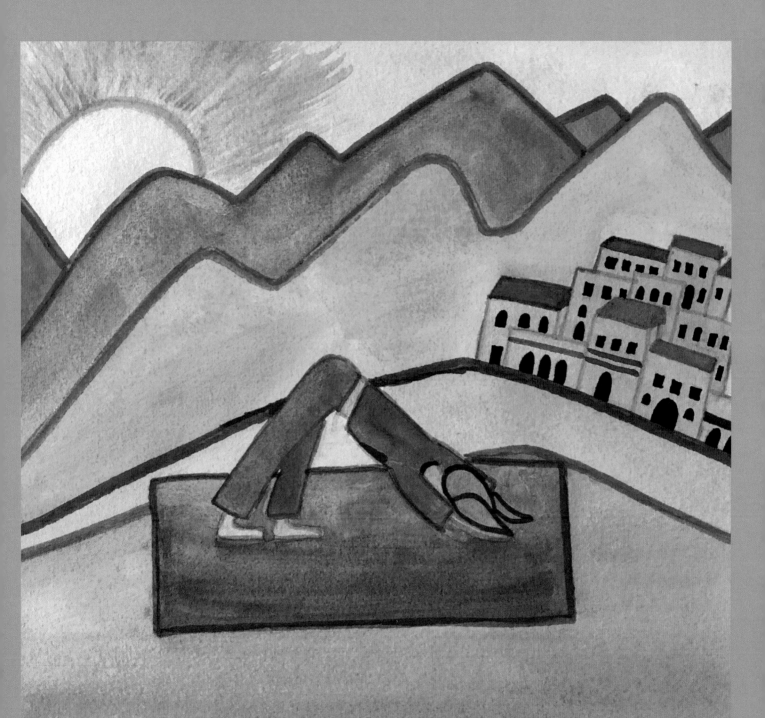

Another animal we may come across in the Amazon Rainforest is the Poison Dart Frog. You will want to stay away from these adorable little frogs, who grow between 1 cm to 6 cm in length. They are one of the Earths most poisonous creatures. They can be found in the trees, on logs and the forest floor. Some of the rainforest trees grow as high as 46 metres.

Yogi Squat/ Malasana to Tree Pose/ Vrksasana
Step your feet out to the edges of your mat and squat down. Place your elbows to your inner thighs and hands at prayer centre, this is your frog position, hold for a few breaths. Then stretch up to be a tree, place one foot above or below your knee and breathe. Squat back down and repeat on the other side.

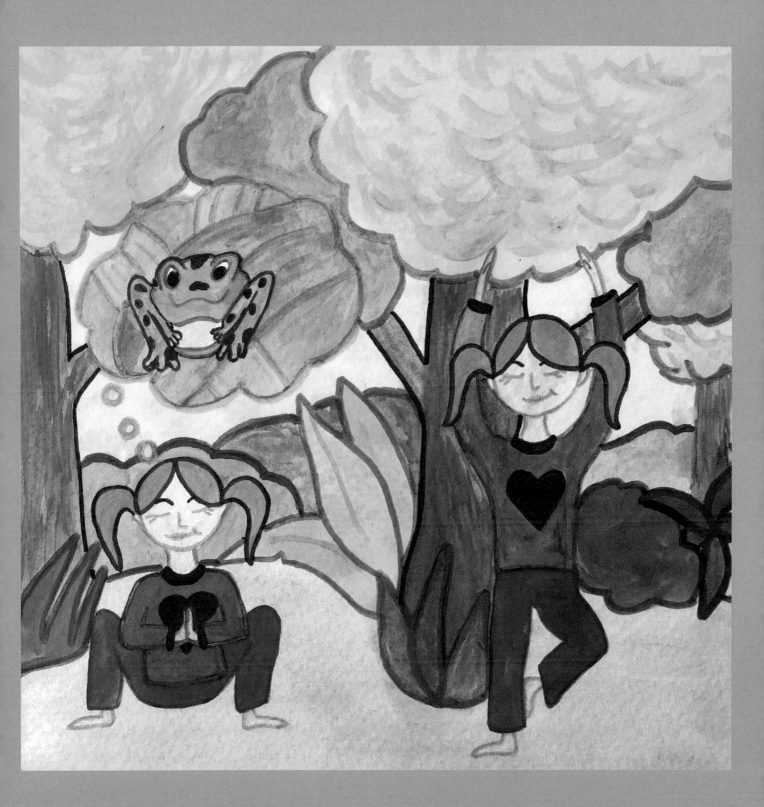

Important news just came in! The Inca treasures have been spotted in the Amazon Rainforest! We can hop on the back of the Andean Condor to fly across the mountain region to the rainforest. The Andean Condor has a wing span of over 3 meters and is the largest flying bird in the world. Even with this large wingspan they can have trouble flying because they can weigh up to 15 kg or 33 pounds.

Warrior III/ Virabhadrasana III
From tree, place both feet on the floor. Breathe in and lift your arms to the sky. Step forward with your rIght foot and lift your left foot and body parallel to the floor. Hold for a few breaths then repeat on the left side.

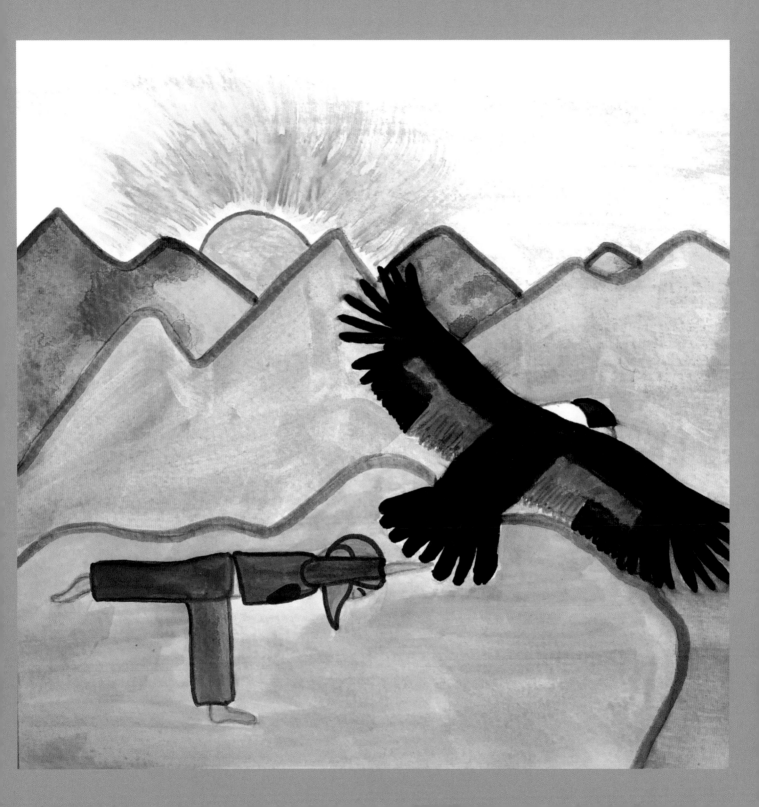

Wow! We landed in the Amazon Rainforest! To say 'thank you' to the Andean Condor for our safe flight, in Spanish we say 'Gracias.' The Amazon is full of dangerous animals. I just spotted an Anaconda! The Green Anaconda is the largest snake in South America. They can grow up to 5 meters or 17 feet in length. There is much folklore and legends about the Anaconda being a mythical shape shifter.

Cobra Pose/ Bhujangasana
From warrior 3 place both feet on the ground and fold forward. Place your hands on the ground and step back into a plank pose. Lower yourself down to your belly. Place your elbows on the mat with your forearms parallel, lift your chest and head towards the sky and breathe.

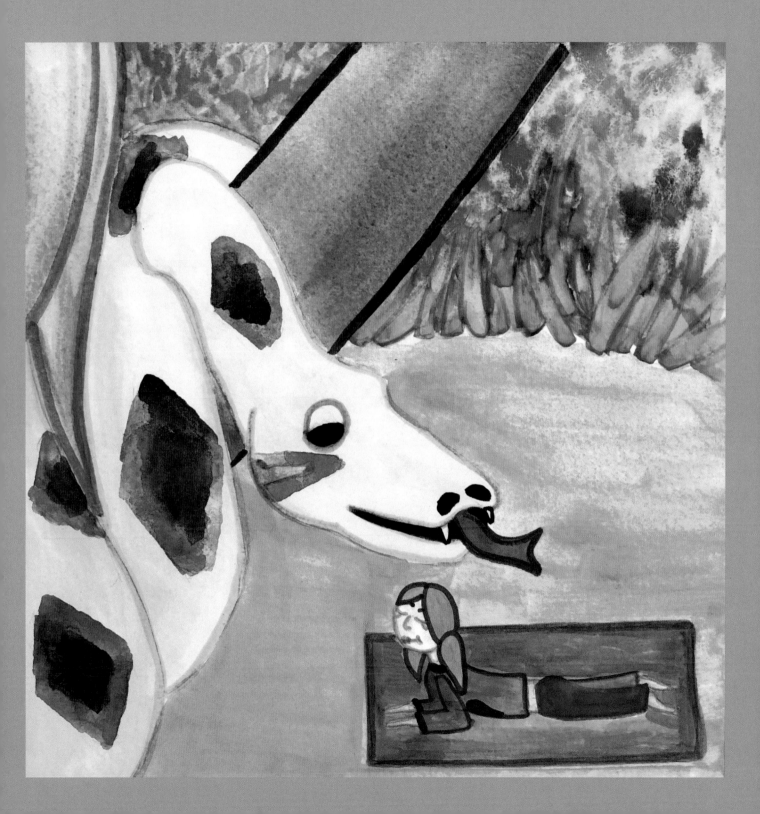

Look over there, I see a spider monkey! Spider monkeys are named after the spider because of the way they hang from the trees with their arms, feet and tails they look like giant spiders. They also are unique because they have virtually no thumb and 4 long fingers. Hmmm I wonder where the treasure could be hiding in the forest. I don't see it anywhere!

Teddy Bear Stand/ Salamba Sirsasana

Come to a kneeling position. Place your hands and head on the floor to make a triangle. Make sure your elbows are bent to create a shelf parallel to the floor. Lift your hips in the air with your toes on the ground, walk your toes towards your torso. Only if you feel balanced lift one knee up and place it on the shelf you have created with your elbow. Again if you feel stable place your other leg on your elbow shelf and balance.

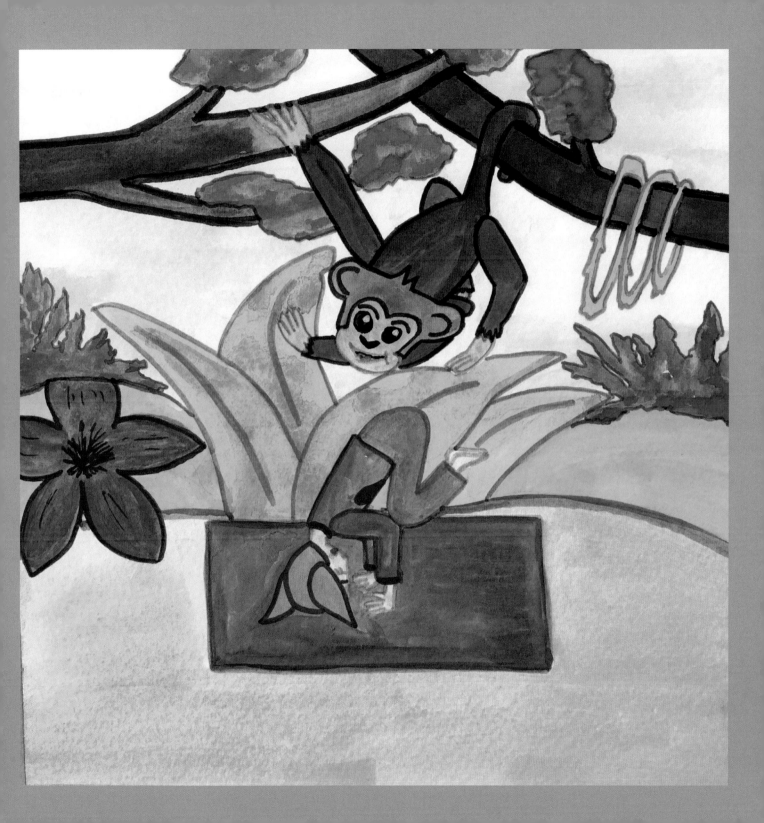

Lets search in the Amazon River. The Amazon River flows through the rainforest and is the worlds largest river, by water volume. Only the Nile is larger when you measure distance. This river is home to the piranha. These fish are known for their sharp teeth, the word piranha translates to "tooth fish" in one of the native Brazilian languages (Brazil is one of Peru's neighbouring countries).

Locust Pose/Salabhasana
Come to your hands and knees and lower yourself to your belly. Place your arms down beside your hips. On an inhale lift your chest, arms and legs while pushing your hips into the floor. Gaze to the top edge of your mat to ensure your neck is an extension of your spine. Hold for 2-3 breaths and then lower down to your belly.

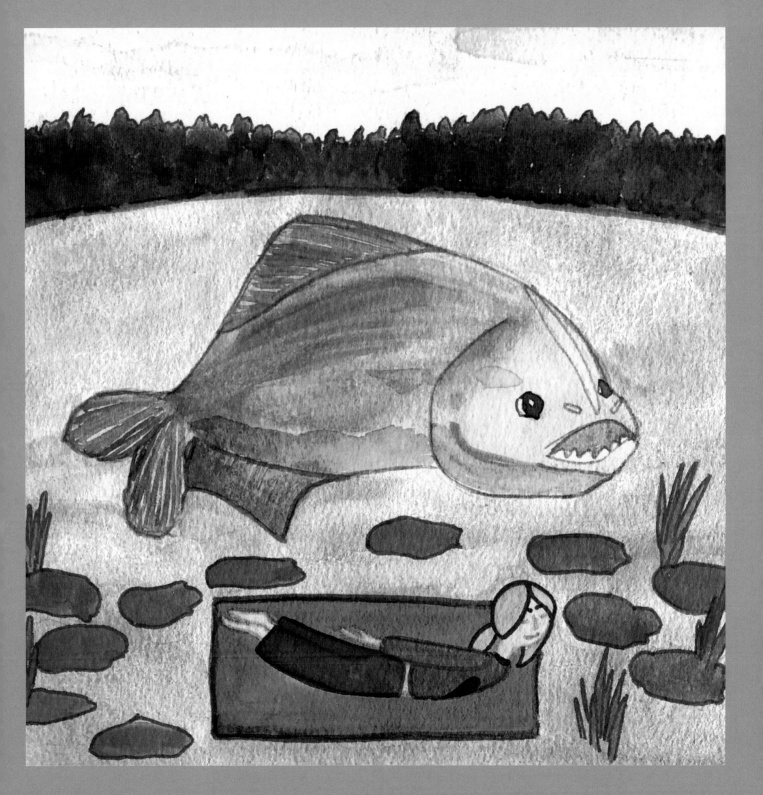

Another unique animal to the river is the Amazon River Dolphin. These dolphins like to feed on piranhas. They are also known as the Pink River Dolphin because of their pale pink colouring and are one of only 3 species of dolphins that live in freshwater. You might want to find these dolphins some glasses because they have really poor eyesight, but don't worry they use their sonar to maneuver through the water.

Dolphin Pose/ Ardha Pincha Mayurasana
Clasp your hands together at the top of your mat, elbows shoulder width apart. Push your hips up to the sky and press your legs straight. Walk your feet towards your elbows.

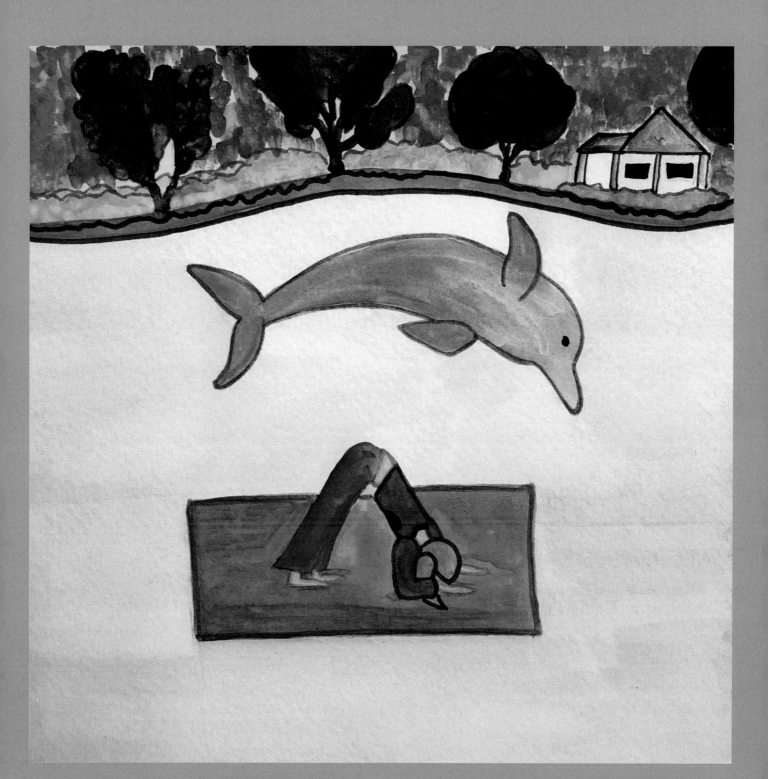

Still no sign of the Inca treasure, wait I see a Scarlet Macaw. The Scarlet Macaw is a beautiful parrot in the Amazon Rainforest. It is known for its colourful plumage and being the largest parrot in the world. He has spotted the Inca treasure on the Island of the Sun or Isla del Sol in Spanish. We will need to fly to the island with the scarlet macaw.

Airplane/ Dekasana

Step to the top of your mat and stand with feet parallel and under hips. Breathe in, focus and stretch your right leg back. Tip forward until you are parallel with the floor. Spread your arms out like wings and fly. Lower your right leg and stand tall. Repeat with your left leg.

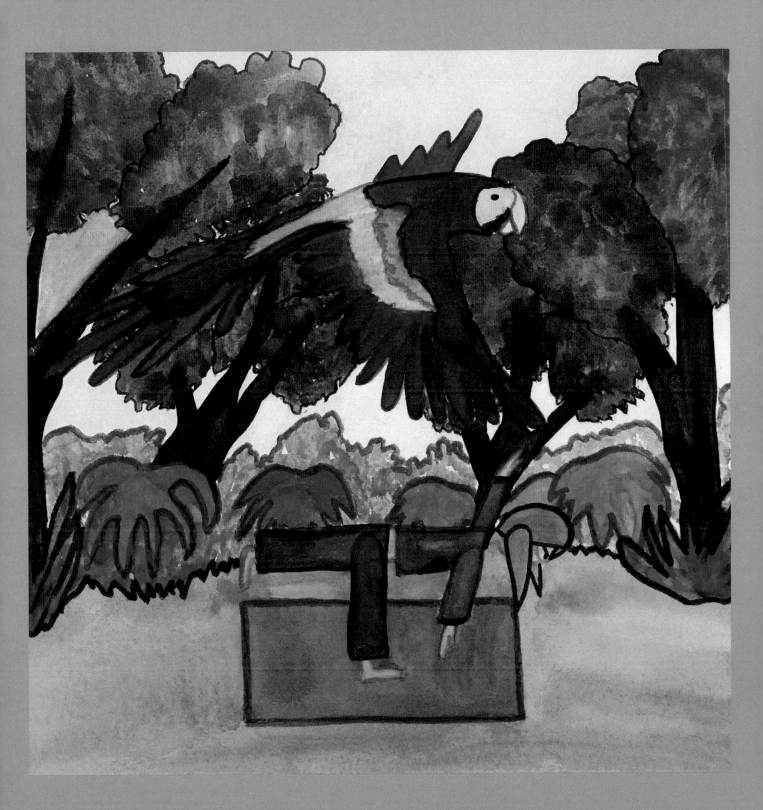

The Island of the Sun is actually located in Bolivia, another neighbouring country to Peru. This island is on Lake Titicaca. Around 800 people live on the island and there are no roads or cars. The ancient Incas believed the Sun God was born on the island, which is why it is called Island of the Sun. There are over 80 ancient ruins on the island that attract many tourists. These thieves are fast they are now headed to the reed islands in Peru.

Warrior I/ Virabhadrasana I
Stand at the top edge of your mat and step your right leg back with your back foot facing the front corner of your mat. Bend your left leg and reach your arms up to the sky. Hold for a few breaths then step forward and repeat with your left leg stepping back. (Your front knee should never bend over your toes if it does widen your stance)

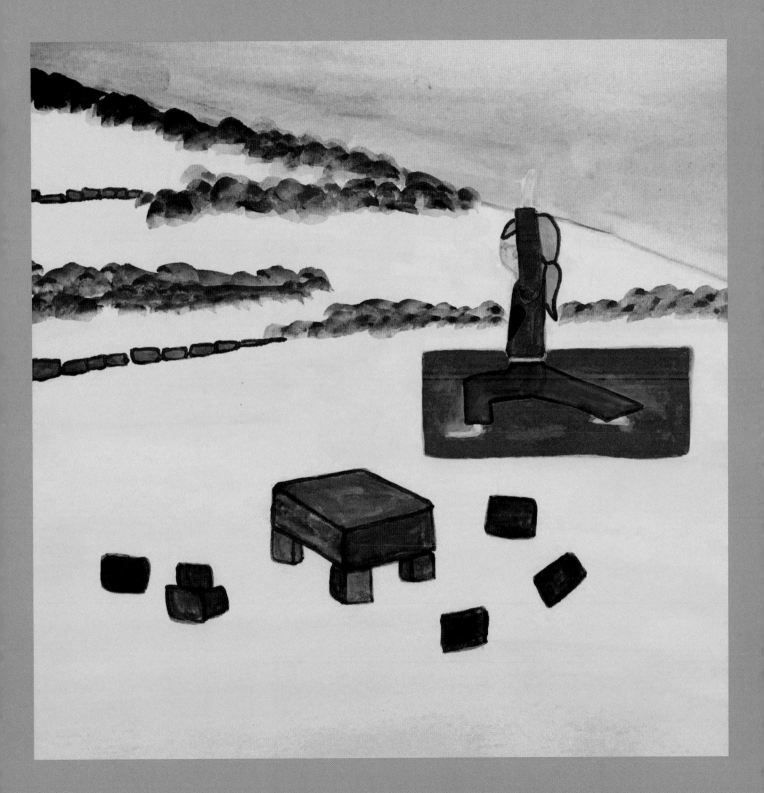

Did you know there are floating islands on Lake Titicaca made completely of totora reeds? There are over 70 of these floating islands made by the Uro tribe. With the expansion of the Incan Empire, the tribe was forced to take up residence on these floating islands 100's of years ago. The reeds are plentiful on the edges of the lake, the Uro's people stack the reeds 4-8 feet thick to make the islands. They place new reeds on the top as the layers below rot.

Boat Pose/ Navasana
Sit on to your bottom with your feet out in front of you, bend your knees in and place your feet on the floor. Put your arms out in front of you and reach for your knees. If you feel supported, lift and point your toes. Hold for 5 breaths.

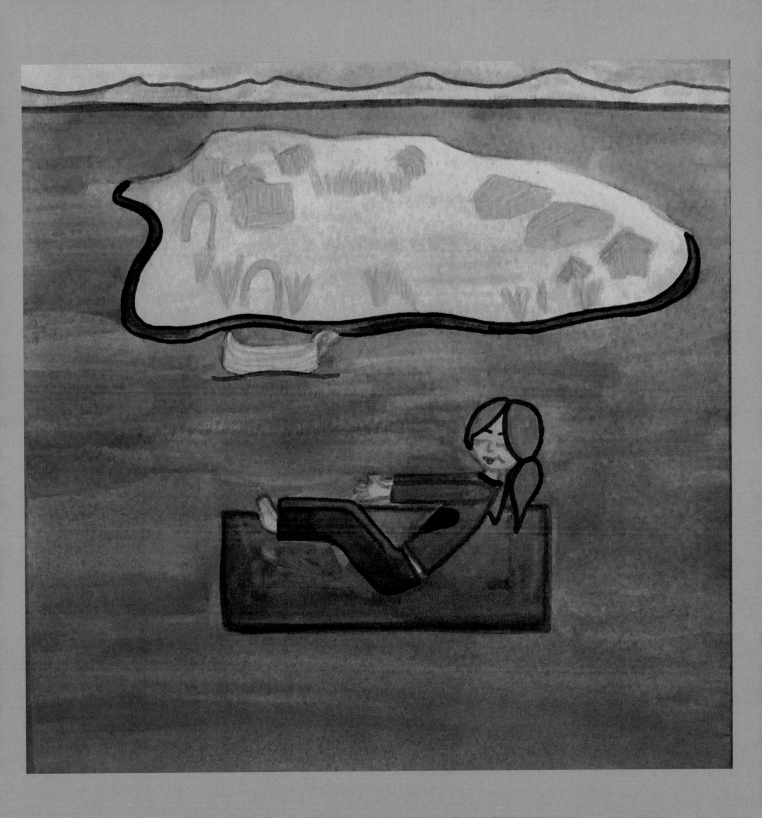

That's it! I know where the treasure is hiding! There is this place known as the Lost City of the Inca's, located deep in the Andes Mountains. I bet the theives will try to hide the treasure there! The Ancient Incas were warriors but they needed to escape the Spanish take over in the 1500's so they retreated into the jungle of the Andes Mountains.

Warrior II/ Virabhadrasana II
Come to standing with feet hip distance apart. Take a step back with your right leg and ensure your heels are in line with each other. Bend your front knee and turn your back foot out to 45 degrees with your toes pointing to the top corner of your mat. Raise your arms to shoulder height and gaze over your left finger tips. Breathe for 5 breaths then step forward and switch legs.

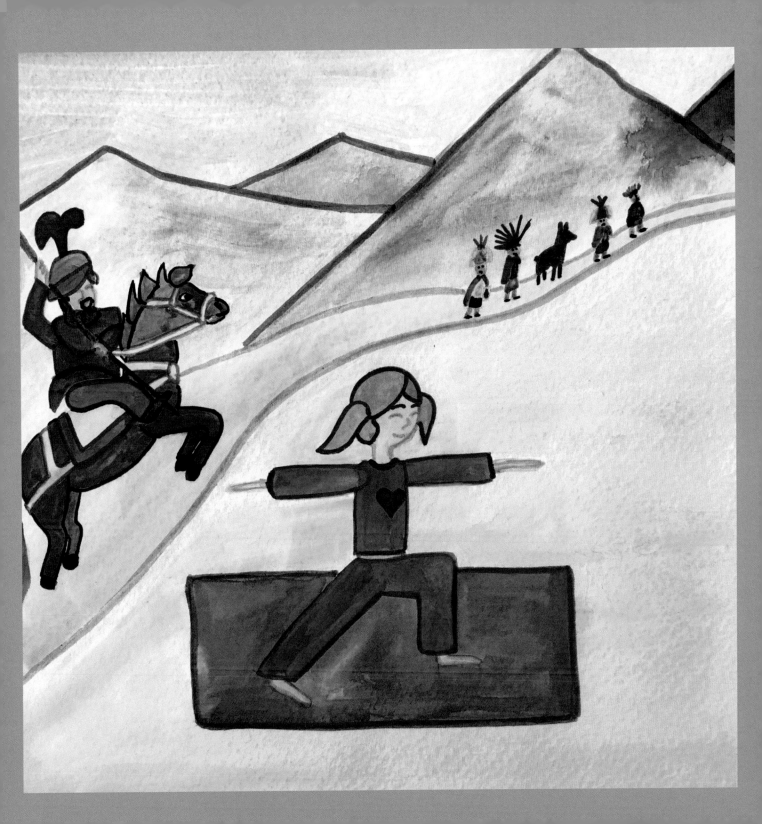

In 1911 this guy named Hiram Bingham III was in search of the Lost City of the Incas called Vilcabamba. While he was searching for it he came across what he thought was Vilcabamba when he rediscovered Machu Picchu. Machu Picchu is now one of the most famous historical sites in the world. In 2007 it was voted one of the New Seven Wonders of the World. Lets check Vicabama first then we can check Machu Picchu!

Humble Warrior/ Baddha Virabhadrasana
From warrior II interlace your fingers behind your back and begin to lean forward over your front foot. As you bow forward ensure that your heart remains open and your front knee does not bend over your toes. Take a few breaths here and repeat on the other side.

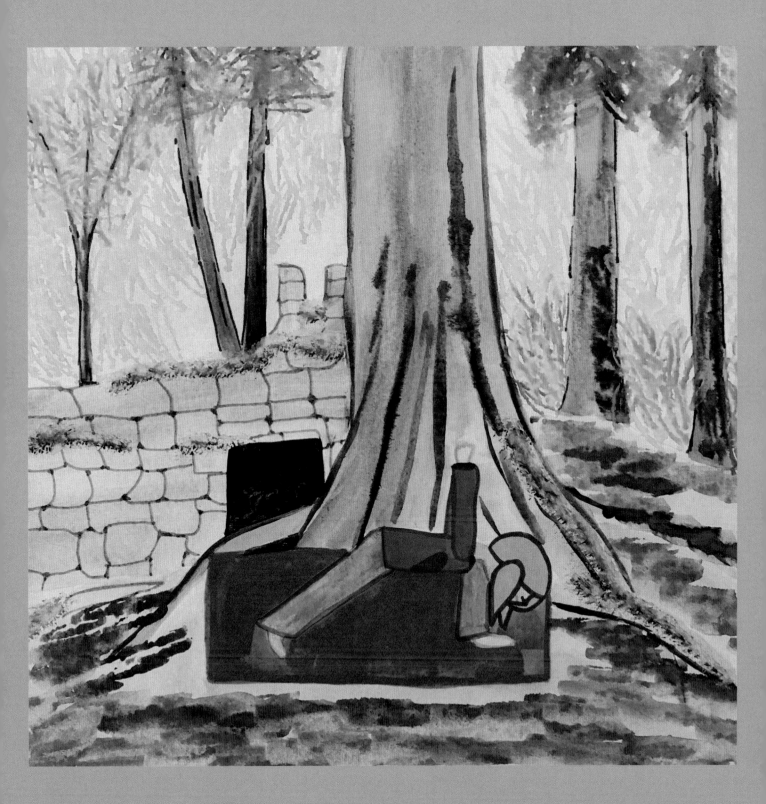

It is not in Vicabama! Machu Picchu is our next best bet! There is a secret temple past Huayna Picchu, each day only the first 400 people to the site are allowed to hike this famous peak. The Incas not only worshiped the sun but the moon as well. On the far side of the Huayna Picchu lookout, there is a trail that will take us there!

Half Moon/ Ardha Chandrasana

Return to Warrior II and place your back hand on your hip. Tilt forward and place your front hand on the floor. Begin to lift your back leg parallel to the floor, rotate your hips to face the wall and strengthen through your legs. If you feel comfortable here begin to straighten your top arm towards the sky. Hold for a few breaths and step back to Warrior II, repeat on the other side.

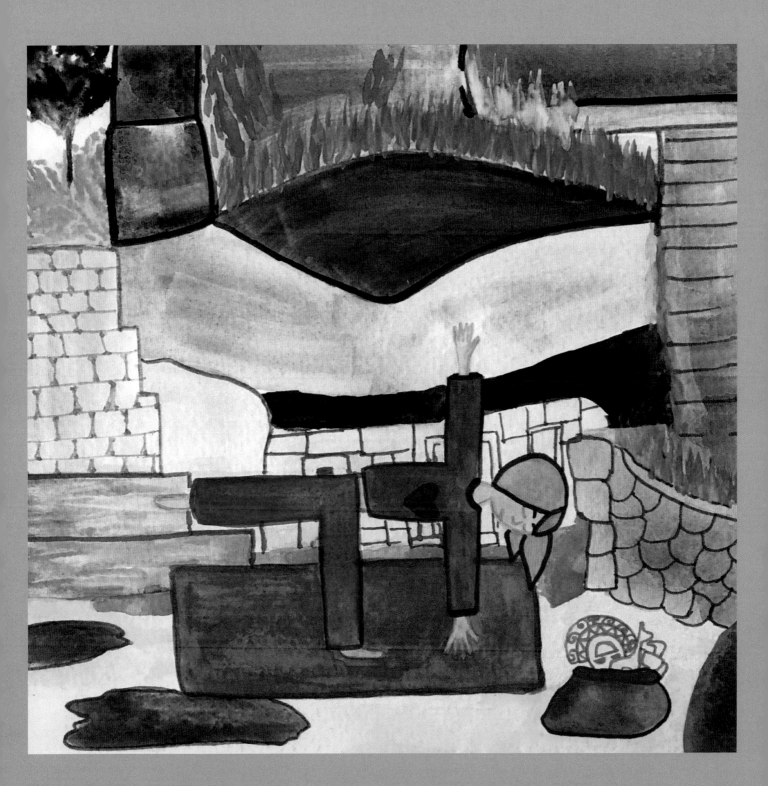

I found the Incan treasure! Now we can return it to the museum. The Incas were very talented gold craftsmen and made many objects out of gold such as masks, sculptures and bowls. Some of these items are priceless as they tell tales of how the Inca's lived. My favourite is the llama sculpture, these were buried with the dead as an offering to the gods to bring abundance to the Incan herds

Standing Forward Fold/ Uttanasana

Step to the top edge of your mat. Take a big inhale then exhale and begin to bend forward from the hips. Emphasize lengthening your front torso as you fold forward. Let your head hang and breath here for 30 seconds.

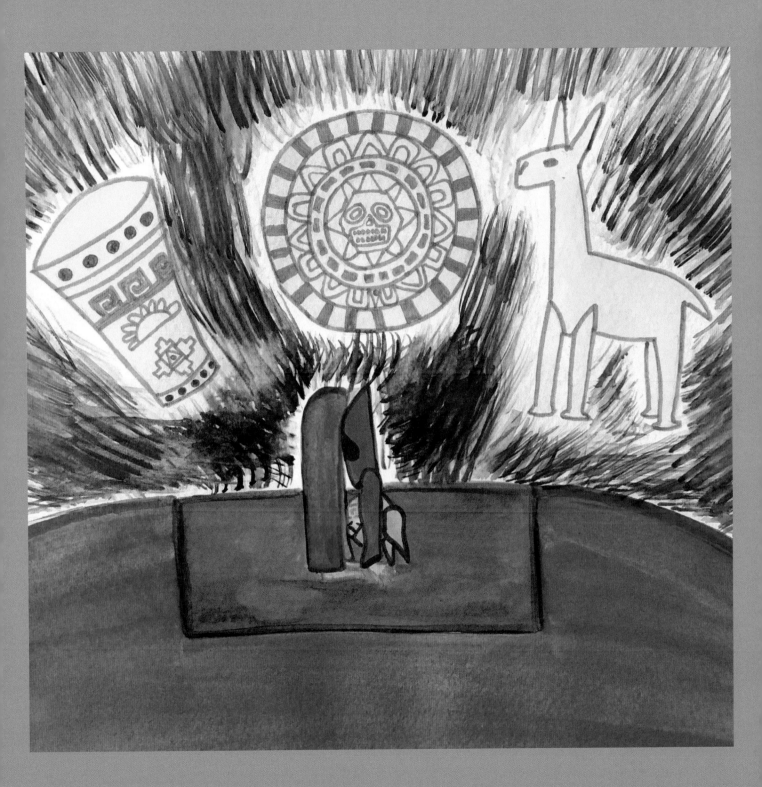

Wow! What a journey we have had across this beautiful country. Standing here looking over the famous Machu Picchu brings about a sense of awe and wonder. No one knows how the Incas build this amazing community hundreds of years ago without the aid of modern machines. I wonder if scientists and archeologists will ever figure out the mysteries of this place.

Mountain Pose/ Tadasana
Bring your hands back to your hips and begin to rise to standing with a flat back. Step your feet together with your big toes touching and heels slightly parted. With your arms at your sides, face your palms forward. Lengthen your spine and stand tall, feel your feet grounding into the earth and breathe.

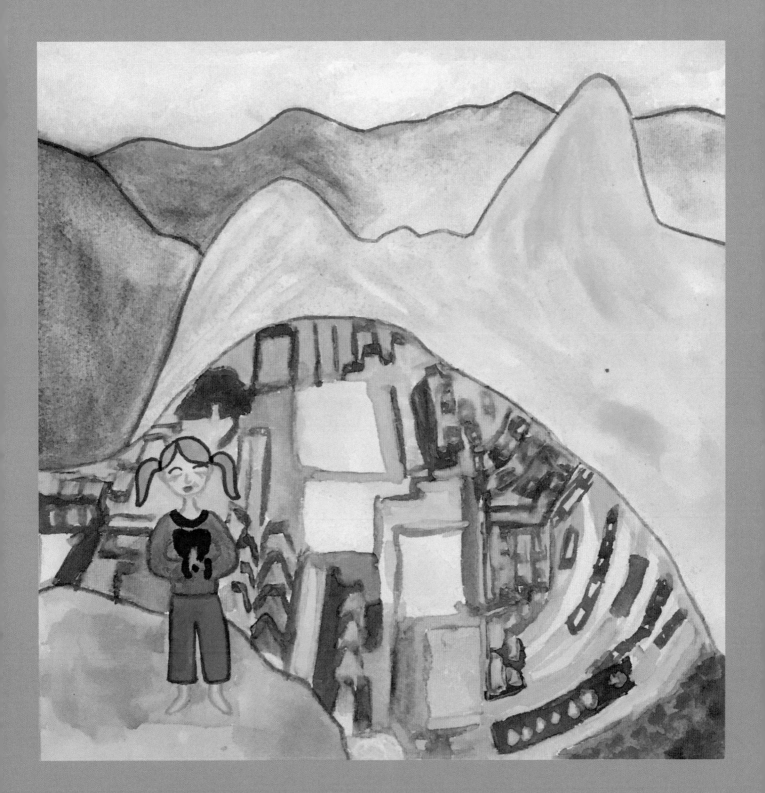

Guided Visualization

Lay down on your mat and begin to imagine that your mat is a log floating on the Amazon River. What would you see? What colours are around you? What sounds would you hear? Visualize your mat as a log gently floating down the river. Noticing any sounds the jungle might make and the gurgling sounds of the slow moving river.

Sit up on your log. What do you see? Notice the Amazon Rainforest surrounding the river. There are many layers to the rainforest. The forest floor is dark and cool as the light from the sun is blocked by the trees and bushes over head. The understory layer is just above the forest floor. Very little sunlight reaches this area either. Plants have to grow very large leaves to collect enough sunlight to survive. Take a moment to notice the large leaves and the hints of sunlight. As you notice this area of the forest you might meet some jaguars, red-eyed tree frogs or leopards. There are alway lots of insects buzzing about this layer of the forest. Take a moment to breath it all in.

Look up slightly higher. You will notice the canopy layer, in this layer the trees have smooth oval shaped leaves that come to a point. It is like a maze of leaves and branches. There are also many animals who live here. Take a moment to breath in and think of the animals you may see. There could be snakes or toucans.

As you look to the top of the forest you notice the emergent layer. The tallest trees are here, they can tower to as high as 200 feet above the forest floor. They are ancient and majestic.

You begin to wonder about the life the trees have had and what they have seen. The trees have huge supportive trunks that are up to 16 feet around. The sunlight is plentiful here. You feel the warm sun on your face and the moist heat that fills the rainforest. Up in the sky you notice some beautiful butterflies and eagles. In the highest branches you also notice some monkeys chattering about and some bats hanging taking a much needed nap.

The rainforest is such an amazing place. As you continue to float down the Amazon River on your log allow your breath to soften with the water, your feet are heavy and fall open to the sides. Notice any tension in your legs, let that go and pour off into the water.

Breathe in lift your chest up and relax your shoulders back onto your mat let your finger tips dip into the water. Relax your jaw and soften your tongue. Feel the warm sun on your forehead, allow the warmth of the sun to release any tension in your head. You are safe, you are left feeling calm, peaceful and so happy. Breathe into this feeling of calm and relaxation and take it with you for the rest of your day. Namaste!

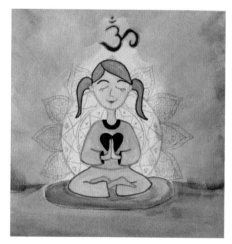

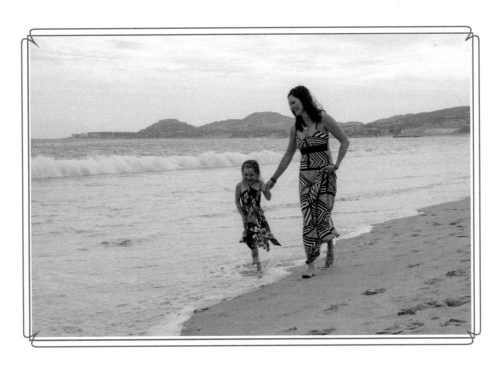

About the Author

Believe, Create, Inspire

Mission is to help people develop and explore their creative gifts through art, yoga and mindfulness. Amanda is an author, illustrator, and teacher (B.A, B.Ed, M.Ed). She lives in Calgary, Alberta with her daughter Ella. Her passions are drawing, creating, yoga and reading. Ella also loves to draw and paint, she even helped her mom with some of the illustrations for this book.

www.artmindfulnessandcreativity.com

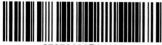

Made in the USA
Columbia, SC
07 October 2018